Table of Contents

What Is Bipolar Disorder?

Historically, persons with bipolar disorder may have been called simply moody or even insane at times. Later, the diagnosis was called manic-depression. While this term is still sometimes used, the generally accepted term is "bipolar disorder".

The two major phases of bipolar disorder are mania and depression. There are other facets of the illness, but they are all aspects of the two. Bipolar disorder is found equally in men and women. About 1 percent of the population can be found to have bipolar disorder.

Mania can be further divided into two categories: hypomania and full-blown mania. Hypomania is simply a state of intense energy and often high productivity. Those who never go beyond this point in bipolar disorder can be great salesmen or high-powered businessmen. The problem is that, for many, full-blown mania is just around the corner.

Full-blown mania tends to have more devastating effects on the person with bipolar disorder. The activity becomes so intense that ventures are undertaken with no actual potential for success, although the person with bipolar disorder cannot see that fact.

There is no consideration for the consequences of actions. Money may be spent which is needed for basic needs. Checks may be written when there is no money in the account. People with bipolar disorder are also often overly generous and give away things that they highly treasure or cannot afford to give away. They tend to regret these gifts later.

The manic state in those with bipolar disorder can be characterized, too, by a gregariousness that is beyond the ordinary out-going person's. This can lead to, among other things, sexual exploits that will cause unwanted results such as pregnancies, disease, or damage to relationships.

The manic phase of bipolar disorder can lead into a period of psychosis. This is marked by bizarre thoughts, such as delusions, or hallucinations. When in a state like this, people with bipolar disorder cannot protect themselves from hazards in their environments because they no longer know what is real.

Usually with mania, eventually there comes depression. The person with bipolar disorder may retreat into seclusion, may even go to bed for days. Sleeping, appetite, and energy level will all be effected.

The gravest danger for the person with bipolar disorder is suicide. All threats should be taken seriously, of course. However, during the depression phase of bipolar disorder they should be especially guarded against.

There has also been a term for those who abuse drugs and alcohol to help them cope with bipolar disorder. This is called "dual diagnosis". It occurs especially in adults and teenagers. These addictions further complicate both the diagnosis and treatment of bipolar disorder. However, it seems to go along with the disease in many instances.

People with bipolar disorder have a wide variety of problems to manage. The reason for optimism is that many have found ways, through medication, therapy, routines, and other methods, to have some degree of control.

People have been having problems such as these for centuries. It is just in modern times that there has been adequate help for the condition. The name for bipolar disorder is newer than the disease, but whatever you call it, its effects can range from the difficult to the deadly. Treatment can be crucial.

About Bipolar Affective Disorder

Bipolar affective disorder, also known as bipolar disorder or manic depression, is a mental illness in which the patient has mood swings or mood cycling. The mood cycles between depression, mania, and normal behaviors. Depression episodes are typically accompanied by extreme sadness and feelings of hopelessness or worthlessness, decreased energy, and sleeping too much. Manic episodes are typically accompanied by extreme happiness, inability to sleep, increased energy, racing thoughts, and distractibility. Mixed episodes, in which the patient shows symptoms of both mania and depression at the same time can also occur.

Bipolar affective disorder is caused by a combination of neurological, biological, emotional, and environmental factors. The true causes of bipolar affective disorder are not fully understood. However, researchers and doctors are continually making advances in this area.

There are two types of bipolar affective disorder. The first type involves an almost constant state of minor mania, with alternating periods of extreme mania and depression. The second type of bipolar affective disorder involves an almost constant state of depression, alternating with small, minor bouts of mania.

Before bipolar affective disorder was fully understood, people with the first type of the illness were often misdiagnosed as schizophrenic. This is due to the fact that many with type one bipolar affective disorder have tendencies to lose touch with reality, have hallucinations, or have delusions during more severe manic phases.

The second type of bipolar affective disorder is often misdiagnosed as clinical depression. This is because the patient is most often depressed, and does not complain about being happy during their manic episodes. The diagnosis is usually corrected after medication treatment has begun for depression. Anti-depressants used with bipolar patients tend to throw the patient into a manic phase. If this happens, the doctor will immediately realize their error and switch the patient to a mood stabilizer.

There are many treatment options for bipolar affective disorder. The most common treatment for bipolar affective disorder is a combination of medication and therapy, or counseling. Medication options include mood stabilizers, anti-depressants, and anti-psychotics. Therapy options include traditional counseling methods, cognitive behavioral therapy, emotive behavioral therapy, and rational behavioral therapy. CBT, EBT, and RBT are fairly new forms of bipolar affective disorder therapy treatments that have been found to be extremely successful. Patients who are not candidates for medication can often have successful results with CBT, EBT, or RBT therapy alone.

While bipolar affective disorder is not a new illness, there is still very little known about the subject. As doctors and researchers learn more about the brain and how it functions, the more likely a cure for bipolar affective disorder will be found. In the meantime, people who feel that they may show symptoms of bipolar affective disorder should contact a mental health professional for diagnosis and treatment options. Family or friends who notice these symptoms in others should also seek to help that person find help for their mental illness. Bipolar affective disorder does not have to control your life, if you are willing to undergo treatment to control it.

The Causes of Bipolar Disorder?

Bipolar disorder is a difficult illness to manage and to treat. Many who have it may ask themselves, "Why me? What caused all this?" There are great disagreements as to the causes of bipolar disorder. They all tend to go back to the old nature/nurture controversy. In other words, does a thing happen to a person because of who he or she is, or because of the environment he or she grew up in?

The nature side of bipolar disorder causes has always been seen in family histories. This, however, can be misleading. Families often pass behaviors on from one generation to the next, regardless of whether family members are natural relatives or adopted ones.

The scientific concept of correlation without causation may account for shared histories of bipolar disorder in biologically unrelated siblings. This concept is easy to grasp. For example, a man could state that all summer, every time he got a sunburn he ate fish. So, did the sunburn cause the man to eat fish? No, but the act of fishing both caused the man's skin to burn and allowed him to catch a fish, which he then ate. In a similar way, bipolar disorder can occur in families without anything in one family member's bipolar disorder causing the bipolar disorder of another.

Also, for whatever reason, people with bipolar disorder are often drawn to each other. In this case it is unclear whether the families formed come together because of their shared genetically similar predisposition towards bipolar disorder, or whether some members of the families are genetically more prone to bipolar disorder but the illness of some other members of the family becomes exaggerated more than it would in another environment.

Research into the genetic causes of bipolar disorder is often done using twin studies. It is assumed that twins will have environments that are as close as is possible. Identical twins are used to show the effects of genetics, since they will share the same genetic materials. Fraternal twins are used as a control group. While these twins share nearly identical environments with their twins, the fraternal twins have less genetic material in common.

It has been shown through these twin studies, and other studies where identical twins are compared to adopted siblings, that there does seem to be a genetic basis for bipolar disorder. Only one percent of the population has bipolar disorder. Fraternal twins, who share some genetic information, are 20 percent more likely to have the disease if one has it. The percentage for identical twins is even higher, at around 60 to 80 percent chance of one having it if the other does.

Environmental causes of bipolar disorder are more difficult to assess. Bipolar disorder has been proven to have a chemical basis in the brain, but the chemical reactions can be caused by any number of factors. A history of losses early in life can be a contributing factor, as can any major source of stress. Physical illnesses such as cancer and others can lead to a depressive state, which is then often followed by mania.

Neither genetics nor environment can fully explain the causes of bipolar disorder. Research is constantly being undertaken in both areas. In the meantime, the nature/nurture controversy is just beginning to heat up.

Symptoms of Bipolar Disorder

From historical figures to celebrities to everyday people, there are many people with bipolar disorder. Whether one hears of these people on television or in real life, the question often arises as to how they know they have bipolar disorder. So, what are the symptoms of bipolar disorder?

Since there are two distinct parts of bipolar disorder, there are also two separate sets of symptoms of bipolar disorder. These symptoms of bipolar disorder many times reflect opposites from the manic to the depressive sides of the illness.

The most obvious of the opposites in the symptoms of bipolar disorder is level of energy and activity. In depression, the person will feel a loss of energy and suffer from fatigue. That person may even appear to be slow. On the other hand, the manic person will have an increased level of energy and much more than usual activity.

Degree of self-esteem is another of the symptoms of bipolar disorder. A depressed person feels unworthy or is guilt-ridden. A manic, though, is so full of him- or herself that he or she has unreasonable ideas of him- or herself or even delusions of grandeur.

This loss of self-esteem may be what leads the depressed person to be indecisive and overblown self-importance that urges the manic to become reckless. Neither the depressed person nor the manic one sees these decision-making processes as symptoms of bipolar disorder. But that is exactly what they are.

The symptoms of bipolar disorder differ from the depressive to the manic mostly because the general themes are different. In depression, everything is slow, dull, small, introverted, and hopeless. In mania, things are overblown, huge, fast, outgoing, and full of impossible dreams.

Some symptoms of bipolar disorder seem, on the surface, to be similar. For example, the poor concentration of the depressed person may appear similar to the distraction of the manic person. They both, in fact, have trouble holding a thought in their heads. This happens for different reasons, though. The depressed person has fewer thoughts but just cannot focus on any, while the manic person has excessive thought and goes rapidly from one to the next.

Sleep cycles vary in both depressed people and manic people. This is one of the symptoms of bipolar disorder which cause trouble for both. The depressed person may not care whether he or she sleeps or not, sometimes sleeping for long periods and sometimes not bothering to go to bed. The manic person will most surely feel little or no need for sleep. He or she may go without sleep for days.

The symptoms of bipolar disorder which vary the most from depressives to manics happen at the far ends of the spectrum. A person who is extremely depressed is likely to think dark thoughts about death, suicide, and even plans to commit suicide. The person who is manic enough can have strange thoughts such as delusions, and bizarre perceptions such as auditory and visual hallucinations.

If a person is truly bipolar, he or she will display some, if not all, of the symptoms of bipolar disorder on both the depressed and manic sides of the line. Because this illness is so serious and can have life changing consequences for the person with it, it is important to recognize the symptoms of bipolar disorder.

A Bipolar Disorder Diagnosis

Living with a bipolar disorder diagnosis isn't easy. However, knowing, as they say, is half the battle. Once a diagnosis is established, a person has two main choices right off. They are whether to let the disorder take control of one's life, or to fight it with every weapon in the modern psychiatric and psychological arsenal.

If fighting for normalcy is the answer, then a bipolar disorder diagnosis can make one aware of what one is fighting. Bipolar disorder can touch every aspect of a person's life, so someone with a bipolar disorder diagnosis will need to be wary on all fronts.

First of all, if there is a bipolar disorder diagnosis then there must have been some sign of the disease. The more severe this manifestation is, the more likely one is to take notice. It is important, though, to treat the illness as soon as a bipolar disorder diagnosis is obtained.

Early treatment can often help prevent some of the more extreme manic highs and depressive lows of bipolar disorder. The earlier treatment is successfully begun, the less the devastating effects of the disease on the person with a bipolar disorder diagnosis.

Early treatment is helpful. The challenge is to keep someone interested in taking medications or engaging in talk therapy when there has been no crisis to set him or her on this path. Such a person needs to be convinced that their bipolar disorder diagnosis is accurate.

For others, the first signs of illness are so overwhelming they consider their bipolar disorder diagnosis to be a relief. For them, it is just good to know that there is a name for what is happening to them and that there are treatments.

For these people, it is extremely important to keep taking medications that are prescribed. This is a responsibility one has to oneself when he or she gets a bipolar disorder diagnosis. If the medication seems to be causing problems, it is important to contact the prescribing doctor to discuss the matter. If no satisfaction can be obtained, finding another doctor is even preferable to simply stopping the medications on one's own.

Those with a bipolar disorder diagnosis usually are given the recommendation to take some form of counseling, or talk therapy. Some may balk at the notion that talking to a therapist can effect their disease. The truth is that these therapies have been shown to have a positive effect on those with bipolar disorder diagnosis.

There are other actions a person with a bipolar disorder diagnosis can take to help lessen their illness. These include the ways a person takes care of him or herself in day to day life. It may seem obvious that a person should eat and sleep in reasonable amounts and times, or do an adequate but reasonable amount of exercise. A person with a bipolar disorder diagnosis will probably find that these common acts do not come naturally. However, with some conscious effort they can begin to see some difference.

A bipolar disorder diagnosis can certainly seem to complicate one's life. It can lead one to take medications, submit him or herself to talk therapy, and take the time and energy to regulate his or her own personal habits. On the other hand, all these concessions to the disease can help a person to live a much calmer and more fulfilling life than that person would had he or she never gotten their bipolar disorder diagnosis. In other words, it doesn't have to be the end of the world.

Recognizing Bipolar Disorder Symptoms

There may come a time when a person needs to determine if a loved one needs to seek help for his or her problems. In fact, there may come a time for many when it is important to be able to recognize bipolar disorder symptoms.

Bipolar disorder symptoms fall into three main categories. These are manic symptoms, psychotic symptoms, and depressive bipolar disorder symptoms. If several of these symptoms are occurring, it may be time to go in for a consultation.

Manic bipolar disorder symptoms are numerous. They all share a certain feeling, though. Everything is faster, grander, and generally bigger than life. A person in a manic state may be much more active than usual. He or she may think and talk faster than he or she usually does. Everything about that person is exaggerated, including his or her overwhelming feeling of self-importance.

Such a person may have grand schemes and adventures in the works. When these plans don't pan out, that person will generally put the blame on some extraneous factor if, in fact, he or she takes the time to consider it at all. Usually, it's simply off to the next idea. These are not just whimsical behaviors, but are actually bipolar disorder symptoms.

When manic, people tend to be reckless. They can end up doing things that effect their personal relationships or may go so far as landing them in jail. This may be seen by someone who is not alert to bipolar disorder symptoms as simply a problem with their conduct. The truth is that those people probably need treatment to do better. It isn't just a matter of making up one's mind to do the right thing.

There are also physical bipolar disorder symptoms of mania that may be quite obvious. A person who feels little or no need for food or sleep may turn out to be in a manic state. While some may be able to function this way, at least for a while, most of us need rest and sustenance to maintain ourselves.

Psychotic bipolar disorder symptoms come mostly with mania, but can come often with mixed moods and occasionally with depressive bipolar disorder symptoms. Psychosis merely refers to a break with reality. This can come in the form of hallucinations, both auditory (hearing voices, etc.) and visual. Delusions, or false beliefs, are also bipolar disorder symptoms. For example, a person may falsely believe that he or she is actually some famous historical figure.

During depression, bipolar disorder symptoms can often be easily seen if one is willing to look carefully. Apathy may be a sign of depression, but other clues are even more telling. Indecisiveness and low self-esteem seem to go hand in hand in depressive bipolar symptoms.

Physical bipolar disorder symptoms of depression include fatigue, weight gain or loss, and eating or sleeping more or less than usual. The person who is displaying bipolar disorder symptoms of depression seems to be telling the world that he or she simply doesn't care enough take good physical care.

One should never look for trouble where there is none. There is no need to be afraid of any slight variation in the moods or habits of a loved one. However, if things just don't seem right, it doesn't hurt to be able to recognize bipolar disorder symptoms.

Psychiatric Evidence of Bipolar Disorder

Bipolar disorder, or manic depression, is a serious mental illness that has eluded doctors for decades. For many years, bipolar disorder patients were diagnosed as psychotic or schizophrenia. However, about twenty years ago, manic depression became a more common diagnosis. Psychiatric specialists still, however, did not really understand the illness.

Over time, more psychiatric evidence has come to light that proves that bipolar disorder, as it is now called, is actually caused by chemical imbalances in the brain. Other factors, both medical and situational, can be involved as well. In the last few years, psychiatric specialists and researchers have determined that bipolar disorder actually has varying degrees of severity, as well as types of symptoms.

Studies of bipolar patients conducted by psychiatric professionals and researchers has long suggested that bipolar disorder runs in families, or, in other words, is hereditary. Through careful study and research of the functions of the brain, it has now been determined how this illness is indeed hereditary and biological in nature.

According to research posted in the American Journal of Psychiatry in 2000, patients with bipolar disorder actually have thirty percent more brain cells of a certain class that have to do with sending signals within the brain. These additional brain cells cause patients' brains to actually behave differently, making them predisposed to have periods of mania or depression.

According to researchers, this type of brain cell regulates moods, how someone responds to stress, and cognitive functions. When the extra brain cells are present, a congestion of cells regulated one type of mood or cognitive function is overloaded, and therefore causes a bout of mania or depression. It is not yet known by psychiatric researchers, however, why patients with bipolar disorder have these additional brain cells. To discover this, more genetic research will be required.

In addition to brain cells and brain chemistry, it has also been speculated by psychiatric researchers that various genes in the genetic makeup of bipolar patients can also contribute to the cause of and hereditary nature of bipolar disorder. Studies have been ongoing experimenting with removal of the gene in mice. The evidence suggests that circadian genes, which regulate mood, hormones, blood pressure, and heart activity may be linked to bipolar disorder. Specifically, the absence or abnormality of the gene actually seems to bring about mania episodes.

All in all, more research needs to be done. Medical and psychiatric researchers and doctors have a lot more to learn about the brain and how it functions. While current treatments seem to work for bipolar disorder, they also have severe side effects. Often, medications prescribed for bipolar disorder have to be monitored, dosages modified, or medications switched entirely for patients to maintain balance. The more we learn about the brain and it's functions, the more we can learn about the physical, biological causes of bipolar disorder. The more we learn about the causes of bipolar disorder, the more likely it will become that effective treatments can be found that offer little side effects and more permanent treatment options for bipolar patients.

Prozac for Bipolar Disorder

Prozac is a medication often prescribed for bipolar disorder, bulimia, and anxiety disorders. The medication is highly effective because it acts as a serotonin inhibitor, which means that it helps balance serotonin levels in the brain. Serotonin levels are responsible for mood stability, depressive states, and control of anxiety, fears, or phobias.

Bipolar disorder, or manic depression, is a mental illness that is caused by a combination of biological, neurological, emotional, and situational factors. The true causes of bipolar disorder are not yet fully understood. However, it is understood that imbalances in the neurotransmitters of the brain, such as serotonin, are partially responsible for the predisposition of bipolar disorder in some patients.

Bulimia is an eating disorder in which the patient eats excessively then purges themselves of the food they have eaten through either vomiting or induced bowel movements. Bulimia is caused by a combination of psychological and emotional factors, and in some cases environmental factors. The emotional factors relating to bulimia are very similar if not identical to factors involved with depression and low self-worth issues, which are connected to serotonin levels in the brain.

Anxiety disorders are thought to be caused by erratic fluctuations in brain chemistry. Anxiety is defined as the intense somewhat debilitating feeling that something horrible is going to happen. Everyone feels anxiety at some point, but typically the normal person has a logical reason to feel anxious. With anxiety disorders, the reason for the anxiety may not be known, or it may not be logical if it is known.

Prozac is an effective treatment for bipolar disorder, bulimia, and anxiety because it controls and balances the serotonin levels in the brain. In bipolar patients, it is often prescribed in conjunction with other medications. Prozac is an effective treatment for depression, but may cause manic episodes to worsen. For this reason, Prozac is generally prescribed along with an anti-psychotic drug that helps tone down manic episodes. Therapy sessions or counseling is also generally a part of treatment.

In bulimia patients, Prozac is often the only prescription given. However, it is combined with treatment of symptoms via counseling and therapy. The idea behind this counseling is to identify why the patient has developed a sense of self-worth, and to allow the patient to learn that what they perceive is not necessarily reality. This is very helpful in bulimia patients who binge and purge as a result of how they perceive their bodies.

Anxiety patients are often prescribed Prozac with great success. Counseling may also be a part of treatment. In therapy sessions, patients may learn techniques to control their anxiety through rationalization of situations that may not at first appear rational. For example, if a patient feels anxiety over a cigarette burning in an ashtray, they can learn techniques to allow their mind to rationalize the situation and understand that there is no real danger of fire, and therefore no reason for the anxiety. These techniques are very successful in conjunction with Prozac for treating anxiety.

Overall, Prozac is an effective treatment for mood disorders. Lithium, it is often considered a miracle drug, helping patients gain stability and normal lives while living with an unstable, unrealistic view of themselves or their surroundings.

Famous People With Bipolar Disorder

There have been many famous people with bipolar disorder, or thought now to have had it based on their lifeworks and stories. There have been so many, in fact, that it is considered by some to be a mark of genius. That may or may not be true, but it is easy to see why the connection in made after a look at the many famous people with bipolar disorder.

Writers have been, and continue to be, some of the great famous people with bipolar disorder. Mark Twain was one such writer. He, like many such writers, was highly functional in his writing. However, he could be depressed-seeming and pessimistic at times. He also had overblown business ideas which. Like many manics' ideas never were accomplished.

Kurt Vonnegut, who wrote the modern classic Slaughterhouse-Five and many other books, and William Faulkner, who created an entire fictional place called Yoknapatawha County as a setting for his novels, were two other famous people with bipolar disorder

Some of the most well-known names in modern history have been thought to have had this disorder. These famous people with bipolar disorder include names such as: Winston Churchill, Abbie Hoffman, Edgar Allen Poe, Beethoven, Van Gogh, Isaac Newton. The world would not have been the same without these and the many other famous people with bipolar disorder.

Some famous people with bipolar disorder have written about the disorder. Most notably, Patty Duke wrote a lengthy book on the subject of her own illness. There have been other famous people with bipolar disorder who have written books about the subject. Kay Redfield Jamison, a psychologist well-known in her field wrote two books, including a memoir and a treatise on the connection between the illness and creativity. Besides these, there have been many other books written by famous people with bipolar disorder about their experiences.

Some famous people with bipolar disorder have been posthumously diagnosed to have had it. Many are current stars and may have actually received the diagnosis from their doctors. Some of these are actresses Linda Hamilton, Margot Kidder, Carrie Fisher, and Patty Duke. Others are musicians such as Kurt Cobain, Ozzy Osbourne, Axel Rose, and Trent Reznor of Nine Inch Nails.

In the past, famous people with bipolar disorder lived very difficult lives. They may not have even known that they had any kind of disorder at all. Many thought the way of mania and depression was just the way of the world.

Now, famous people with bipolar disorder are under an extraordinary amount of pressure to work through their cycles of mania and depression. The case of Kurt Cobain proved that bipolar disorder untreated is a disaster. On the other hand, many feel that the medications stunt their creativity. Therapy is seen by some as a vent by which the powerful force of their expression is lost.

This is a controversial topic, and many doctors feel that great strides have been made in medications that are not as debilitating to the creative person. Therapy, too, has changed in many quarters. One thing is certain. The prognosis is better these days than it ever has been for famous people with bipolar disorder.

Bipolar Disorder in Children

Bipolar disorder is a being diagnosed in children as young as six years old in recent years. Some doctors think this is a good assessment of many children while others think the diagnosis is overdone. While it may be just an intellectual controversy to some, others who know a child who may have bipolar disorder will not be amused. It is important therefore to take into account all the facets of the disorder.

It is a tricky diagnosis to say the least. Bipolar disorder in children often appears similar to ADHD, or as simply rambunctious childhood behavior. Young children may cycle fast, meaning that they go from a depressed state to a manic state and back, etc. very quickly, often within weeks or even days.

Suicide attempts often happen on the spur of the moment, with little or no warning. This is different than in most adults where the depression is often long-lasting and suicide attempts may be well thought-out. For this reason it is imperative that children with the disorder be treated successfully.

Bipolar disorder in children often presents in mania. In the younger children this is often likely to come with hallucinations, both auditory and visual. It may seem that these would be difficult to distinguish from a healthy imagination. Sometimes, in fact, it is. Many times, though, the visions and voices are more disturbing and threatening than a healthy child would imagine.

Teens with bipolar disorder are, for the most part, similar in their symptoms to adults. A major complicating factor with teens is the use of drugs and alcohol. As with adults, this practice of trying to use street drugs and alcohol to control mood swings, is called "self-medicating." It is a dangerous business and often masks the symptoms of the disorder. Bipolar disorder in children should always be considered when drugs are being used by them, if only to rule it out.

Bipolar disorder in children who are older, such as teenagers, is still different from the adult disorder in that the person with the disorder is still a minor. This leads to situations where the older child has an adversarial relationship with authorities and is therefore hard to convince that treatment is a good thing.

There are some ways to cut down on the confusion. Speaking with the child's teachers gives an outside opinion of how the child is doing day-to-day. Also, this shows how the child fares in a different setting from the home environment. Bipolar disorder in children, if it is masquerading as some other form of disorder or behavior, is more likely to be found out if more people are alert to its symptoms.

Getting a second opinion is also very important, since so many doctors disagree on bipolar disorder in children. Once the second opinion is obtained, the family can make a more informed decision as to what the problem is and how to proceed. Doctors may not all agree on bipolar disorder in children, but a second opinion should help to clarify the situation. The parent or guardian can listen carefully and determine if the doctor's explanation sounds accurate. Then, ultimately, it is the parents' job to make the call. Misdiagnosis and wrong treatment would be unthinkable, but if bipolar disorder in children is the correct diagnosis, it is surely better to accept it.

Exploring the Various Bipolar Disorders

Bipolar disorders are not all alike. There are even specialized categories for the bipolar disorders which doctors use to distinguish one kind from another. This makes it easier for them to discuss the particular types of problems a patient might be having. A fairly benign and often overlooked member of the family of bipolar disorders is hypomania. It is overlooked for good reason. It is seldom a problem for the person who has it. It may even increase his chances for success by making him more outgoing, quick thinking, and optimistic. Treatment is rarely sought and seldom needed.

The most common disorder to be thought of as one of the bipolar disorders is bipolar I. This encompasses all those who suffer from alternating manic and depressed states. Those with bipolar I go from having the highest opinion of themselves to having little regard for their own well-being. They go from periods of fast and outlandish activity to times of desperation and thoughts of death.

Of all the bipolar disorders, bipolar I is perhaps the most difficult to treat. Mood stabilizers such as lithium or anticonvulsants are useful. If depression, or especially mania, turns into psychosis, an antipsychotic medication is called for to bring the patient back to reality.

The difficulty comes in treating simple depression in bipolar I. An antidepressant would seem to be in order but, for the person who may become manic, it may be dangerous. It could start a cycle of rapid changes from depression to mania and back again in relatively short order. In the bipolar disorders this problem is most prevalent in bipolar I.

Dual diagnosis is another of the bipolar disorders. This is the combination of any bipolar disorder with alcohol and/or drug abuse. Most often, the abuse, in this case, of alcohol or drugs comes after the onset of one of the bipolar disorders.

These substances are used by the person with bipolar disorder to alleviate the symptoms of the illness. A stimulant may seem to help a person to overcome depression, and a depressant, such as alcohol may be thought to lessen the over activity of mania, for example. In reality, the abuse of drugs and/or alcohol only makes the episodes more severe in the end. This is not an answer for those with bipolar disorders.

Less obvious, but also considered one of the bipolar disorders is MDD, or major depression. People with MDD spend most of the time that they are ill being depressed. They may have minor and short manic episodes, but the depression dominates. For these people, life is grim, unsatisfying, and perhaps seems unbearable. Episodes of depression for these people may last for months or sometimes years.

Treatment for these people is usually less complicated. They may respond well to antidepressants, talk therapy, and even to something as simple as exercise. There is less chance of triggering a manic episode, so treatment is less risky in these bipolar disorders.

There are many bipolar disorders. There are also many ways to treat these bipolar disorders. The trick is to match a disorder to the correct treatment and to encourage the patient to follow that treatment to the best of his or her ability. Having words to describe the different bipolar disorders makes it that much easier for the doctors and others to do their parts.

About Type 1 Bipolar Disorder

Bipolar disorder, also known as manic depression, is a mental illness caused by a number of factors including neurological, biological, emotional, and environmental factors. It is typically characterized as mood cycling from manic, or extra happy, moods to depressed, or extra sad, moods.

Many people are not aware that in the last few years doctors have begun diagnosing bipolar disorder as two different types, based on how the moods cycle in the patient. Bipolar disorder type 1, also known as raging bipolar disorder, is diagnosed when the patient has at least one manic episode lasting at least one week or longer. Bipolar disorder type two, also known as rapid cycling bipolar disorder, is diagnosed when the patient has at least one manic episode and one depressive episode within four days to one week.

Hypomania is a severe form of mania that typically occurs in bipolar disorder type 1 patients. This state occurs because the patient is almost constantly up; the normal state for the patient is 1 of mania. Therefore, mood cycling in bipolar disorder type 1 patients often involves mania combined with the mood change. Mania combined with mania creates hypomania. Hypomania also can be accompanied by psychotic symptoms such as the patient becoming delusional or having hallucinations. This is a very simplistic way to describe how hypomania and mixed episodes occur.

Mixed episodes also often occur with bipolar disorder type 1. A mixed episode is hard to explain to the general public. It consists of being both happy and sad, up and down, all at the same time. Generally, this translates into the patient being very depressed emotionally, but displaying symptoms of mania such as inability to concentrate and lack of sleep.

Bipolar disorder type 1 is the most common type of bipolar disorder, and the most treatable. Because bipolar disorder type 1 typically manifests itself in the form of long manic periods with possibly one or two short depressive periods each year, treatment options are much simpler. Since mania requires one type of medication and depression requires another type of medication, the ability to treat only mania makes finding effective medications a much simpler task. Mood stabilizers are also quite effective with type 1 bipolar disorder, without the use of mania or depression medications.

The symptoms that the bipolar disorder type 1 patient experiences determine the type of mania medication used to control the excessive moods. In cases of mild but constant mania, lithium is the drug of choice. However, in cases in which mixed mania or hypomania are consistently present, a stronger drug or anti-psychotic, such as Depakote, is typically prescribed.

Bipolar type 1 is also the likeliest candidate for treatment via Cognitive Behavioral Therapy (CBT). This is because the patient is most often in a state that allows them to easily focus their mind on rationalizing situations, recognizing triggers, and suppressing severe episodes. However, when the patient displays symptoms of hypomania, as some bipolar type 1 patients often do, cognitive behavioral therapy is not as effective during these episodes.

Overall, bipolar disorder type 1 is easily controlled through appropriate treatment and medications. If you experience any symptoms of bipolar disorder type 1 you should contact your doctor to make arrangements for diagnostic testing and to discuss treatment options. Ultimately, the patient is responsible for their own illness, and therefore, their own treatment.

About Bipolar II Disorder

Bipolar disorder is also known as manic depressive disorder. It is a mental illness that presents itself as mood swings or mood cycling. Many people do not realize that there are actually two types of bipolar disorder. Bipolar I disorder is typically defined as raging mood cycling with episodes of extreme mania and depression, as well as the occasional mixed episode. Bipolar I patients may also experience psychotic or hallucinating symptoms.

Bipolar II disorder is typically defined as rapid mood cycling with episodes of hypomania and depression. Bipolar II disorder does not occur with psychotic or hallucinating symptoms. Additionally, hypomania is defined as a milder form of mania, in which the patient has a period of heightened happiness or elation. Depression with bipolar II patients is often more severe than in patients with bipolar I disorder. Suicide, suicide threats, suicide attempts, and thoughts of suicide are much more common in bipolar II patients than bipolar I patients.

A diagnosis of bipolar II disorder is typically made when the patient has had one or more major depressive episodes, at least one hypomania episode, no manic episodes, and when no other reason for symptoms can be found.

Symptoms of depression with bipolar II disorder include decreased energy, unexplained weight changes, feelings of despair, increased irritability, and uncontrollable crying. Symptoms of hypomania include sleeplessness, racing thoughts, distractibility, excess energy, and rash judgments. These symptoms are similar to mania, but are less severe.

Treatment of bipolar II disorder typically involves a combination of medication and therapy or counseling. Medications typically prescribed for treatment of bipolar II disorder include anti-depressants such as Celexa, as well as mood stabilizers such as Topomax. Mood stabilizers are vitally important in treatment of bipolar disorders, because antidepressants alone can cause the patient to enter into a manic or hypomania episode.

Bipolar II disorder is actually often misdiagnosed as clinical depression. This is due to the fact that depression is most often present, and hypomania episodes rarely come to light in therapy sessions due to their upbeat nature. It is typically through treatment by antidepressants that the correct diagnosis is made, because the patient will spin into a hypomania episode almost immediately if the diagnosis should be bipolar II disorder rather than clinical depression.

Counseling or therapy treatment options for bipolar II disorder may include traditional counseling methods, discussion of triggers and life style changes that can lessen the severity of episodes, and cognitive behavioral therapy. Patients with a mild case of bipolar II disorder may benefit from counseling or therapy alone without medication. However, this is less common with bipolar II disorder than with bipolar I disorder, due to the nature of the severity of the depressive states.

It is vitally important for people with symptoms of bipolar II disorder to seek the help of mental health professionals as soon as symptoms become evident. Bipolar II disorder patients account for at least half of the suicides each year. To prevent suicidal behavior, it is important for bipolar II patients to be properly diagnosed at an early stage.

Concerns of Bipolar Disorder Self Injury

In bipolar disorder, there is sometimes concern about bipolar disorder self-injury. This can take many shapes, but is always serious.

One form of bipolar disorder self-injury that is coming most recently into the public consciousness is self-mutilation, or "cutting". This practice is found in people with other diagnoses, too. Bipolar people are just some of those who self-injure.

Cutting, burning or other self-harming behaviors are often seen in adolescent girls and others, even in men. Much of this is a part of bipolar disorder self-injury.

Although people who self-mutilate are often depressed or beyond that, suicidal, these acts are not intended as suicide attempts. They are often desperate acts of those who feel out of control, worthless, or angry. It is no wonder, given the similar symptoms, that this is often a case of bipolar disorder self-injury.

Suicide, of course, is the most extreme form of bipolar disorder self-injury. Before suicide, there may be suicidal ideations, plans for suicide, and possibly many attempts before suicide is committed, if it ever is. In any case, all threats of bipolar disorder self-injury should be taken seriously.

Suicidal thoughts may cloud the thinking of a depressed person to the extent that he or she can think of nothing else. It may seem that the world would be better off without them, or that they can show others that they should have been treated better. At this stage there is concern of bipolar disorder self-injury, but the ideas are just at a simmer.

When a person begins to make plans, the danger of bipolar disorder self-injury becomes more imminent. A person may make elaborate plans for years. Another person may only think of a plausible way to go about it. The trouble is that either of these people may at any time actually commit suicide. It is never easy to predict the likelihood of bipolar disorder self-injury.

Many times a person's suicidal tendencies will not be noted unless an attempt is made. While some attempts seem more serious than others, a wise person will treat all attempts seriously. More serious attempts could be those where a note was found, or the outcome was more certain in comparison to other sorts of attempts. Bipolar disorder self-injury is always possible in these situations.

Whatever the method of attempt at bipolar disorder self-injury, there is seriousness attached to it. After all, people who have attempted suicide in the past are 40 times more likely to commit suicide than those who never have attempted it before.

If a person begins to make final arrangements, or to set his or her affairs in order for no particular reason, suicide may be on his or her mind. It could be as simple as giving away possessions, or as complex as making financial arrangements. If this is suddenly seen in a bipolar individual, it should be determined whether or not that person is in danger of bipolar disorder self-injury.

Many thoughts, plans, or attempts actually do end in suicide. 11 percent of deaths in the US are as a result of suicide. More women than men attempt suicide, but 80 percent of the deaths by suicide are by males. More and more adolescents are committing suicide every year. Bipolar disorder self-injury, then, is a distinct and growing problem.

It is difficult enough dealing with the affective, social, legal, and physical consequences of the disease. Self-harm and suicide makes attention to bipolar disorder self-injury most necessary.

Borderline Personality Disorder VS Bipolar

Borderline personality disorder and bipolar are often mistaken as being the same thing. They are also often misdiagnosed, one for the other. This is because the symptoms for both illnesses are startlingly similar.

Borderline personality disorder is actually less common and less known than bipolar. Borderline personality disorder accounts for only about twenty percent of hospitalizations for mental illness each year, while bipolar accounts for about fifty percent of hospitalizations. Borderline personality disorder is most common in young women, whereas bipolar is equally common in both men and women, as well as all age groups.

Borderline personality disorder and bipolar patients both experience mood swings that may involve violent outbursts, depression, or anxiety. However, while bipolar patients typically cycle through these moods over a period of weeks or months, borderline personality disorder patients may have bursts of these moods lasting only a few hours or a day.

Borderline personality disorder patients also undergo periods of having no idea who they are in terms of personality, likes, dislikes, and preferences. They may change long term goals frequently, and have trouble sticking to any one activity. Acting with impulsiveness, going on major unaffordable shopping sprees, excessive eating, or engaging in risky sexual relationships can also be experienced. These are also symptoms of mania in bipolar patients.

Borderline personality disorder patients may also undergo periods of worthlessness, feeling mistreated or misunderstood, and emptiness. These symptoms coincide with symptoms of depression in bipolar patients.

Another symptom of borderline personality disorder involves how they deal with relationships. Relationships are often viewed in extremes. Either the patient is totally in love or hates with a passion. A patient may be completely in love one minute, then hate someone totally due to a small conflict or situation. Fears of abandonment often lead to suicide threats, rejection, and depression in the patient. These relationship issues can also be found in bipolar patients.

Treatments of borderline personality disorder and bipolar are similar. A combination of therapy and medication is typically preferred by the psychiatrist. Cognitive behavioral therapy, while successfully implemented with bipolar patients, was originally developed for use with borderline personality disorder. Various medications can also be prescribed for either mental illness with successful results.

Like bipolar disorder, little is known about the actual causes of borderline personality disorder. There is a lot of controversy about genetics versus environment in this area. However, it appears through research that, while bipolar is definitely hereditary and biological in nature, borderline personality disorder is more likely to be a result of environment and situational stimuli.

As you can see, many similarities exist between bipolar and borderline personality disorder. It can often be quite difficult to distinguish one illness from the other, even for doctors and psychologists. If you suffer any of the symptoms discussed here, it is important to obtain the assistance and diagnosis of a licensed professional for appropriate diagnosis and treatment of your symptoms. You should never attempt self-diagnosis and treatment for symptoms such as those associated with bipolar and borderline personality disorder without the help of a psychiatrist or psychologist. Doing so may cause your symptoms to worsen, and make treatment less successful in the future.

Celexa and Bipolar Disorder

Bipolar disorder, or manic depression, is a mental illness that manifests itself as mood swings or mood cycling between depressed, manic, or normal moods. There are two types of bipolar disorder. The first type, sometimes called raging bipolar, manifests itself as almost constant mild mania, with periods of sever mania alternating with depression. Mixed episodes where the patient displays both manic and depressive symptoms at the same time can also occur with this type of bipolar disorder.

The second type, sometimes called rapid cycling bipolar, manifests itself as almost constant depression, with alternating periods of mania and severe depression that can often last a few hours or a few days before cycling to the next episode.

Depression symptoms include oversleeping, extreme sadness, feelings of worthlessness or despair, irritability, anger, and withdrawal. Manic symptoms include sleeplessness, increased energy levels, distractibility, racing thoughts, obsessive behaviors, and extreme happiness.

There are many treatment options for bipolar disorder. Most patients with bipolar disorder require a combination of medication and therapy or counseling for successful treatment of symptoms. However, minor cases of bipolar disorder may not require medication, but may require instead cognitive behavioral therapy. There are some cases, such as in patients with a history of drug abuse, where medication may be recommended but is not a viable treatment option. These cases typically also use cognitive behavioral therapy to assist patients in coping with their illness.

Celexa is an anti-depressant, commonly used with bipolar patients. Celexa, or citalopram, is a serotonin reuptake inhibitor, or SSRI. This family of medications has the effect of balancing serotonin levels in the brain, which are thought to be responsible for mood stabilization.

Celexa is most successful as a treatment for unipolar depression and bipolar disorder type two patients. This is because it is an anti-depressant. Serotonin, the chemical in the brain that balances moods and particularly controls strong emotions, often presents imbalances in the form of depression. Celexa corrects these imbalances, giving the patient relief from depression.

Celexa is most successful as a treatment for bipolar disorder type one patients when used in combination with a mood stabilizer. As an anti-depressant, Celexa alone causes bipolar disorder type one patients to swing into a manic episode. Used in combination with a mood stabilizer or anti-psychotic, however, can allow for a balance of moods to take place, ending rapid or raging mood cycling.

Celexa has several possible minor side effects when used for treatment of bipolar disorder. Common side effects include drowsiness, cotton mouth, nausea, and trouble sleeping. Less common side effects include abdominal pain, anxiety, gas, headache, heartburn, increased sweating, pain in muscles or joints, increases or decreases in weight, weakness, and vomiting. If these side effects persist or become unbearable, you should contact your doctor.

Celexa can also have several possible major side effects when used for treatment of bipolar disorder. Common major side effects include a decrease in sexual desire or ability. Less common major side effects include agitation, confusion, blurred vision, fever, increase in urinal frequency, lack of emotion, decreased memory, skin rashes, and trouble breathing. If you experience any of these side effects, you should contact your doctor immediately.

Friends, family and patients with bipolar disorder should keep in mind that even when using anti-depressants such as Celexa, suicide, suicide threats, and suicide attempts can still occur. Always be aware of the signs that can lead to suicide so that medical treatment can be found before an attempt is made.

Bipolar disorder should, in all cases, be treated with a combination of Celexa, or other medications, in conjunction with therapy or counseling. Bipolar disorder patients are encouraged to take active part in their treatment plans. Additionally bipolar patients should not attempt to self-medicate or treat symptoms with medication alone. If you show symptoms of bipolar disorder, you should contact your doctor about Celexa and other treatment options.

Pediatric Bipolar Vs. Asperger's Disorder

Pediatric bipolar disorder, or manic depression, is a mental illness that presents itself in patients as mood swings or mood cycling. Pediatric bipolar type one patients tend to experience episodes of mania alternating with periodic episodes of depression. Pediatric bipolar type two patients tend to experience episodes of depression interspersed with periodic episodes of mild mania. Depression symptoms include anger, extreme sadness, sleeping too much, and feelings of worthlessness. Manic symptoms include bursts of rage, extreme happiness, increased energy, hyperactivity, distractibility, sleeping too little, and obsessive behaviors.

Pediatric bipolar disorder is caused by a combination of neurological, biological, emotional, and environmental factors. Not all factors are present in every case, although most cases include biological and environmental factors. Little is known about the exact causes of pediatric bipolar disorder. However, advances are being made in this area.

Asperger's disorder can be described as a mild form of autism. Actually, Asperger's disorder is a type of pervasive development disorder that can cause developmental issues, especially in the areas of communication and social development. Symptoms of Asperger's disorder include problems with social skills, odd or repetitive behavior or habits, communication difficulties, and obsession with a limited range of interests.

The causes of Asperger's disorder are not yet known. Studies show that Asperger's disorder tends to run in families, meaning that it is hereditary. This fact shows that the underlying cause of Asperger's disorder must be biological, meaning that it is either genetic or neurologically related.

Pediatric bipolar disorder can be misdiagnosed as Asperger's disorder because pediatric bipolar disorder can present itself via symptoms such as obsessive compulsive behavior, odd habits, and bouts of rage. Patients of pediatric bipolar disorder and Asperger's disorder both have symptoms that lead to lacking social development skills, educational issues, behavioral issues, and anger issues.

Pediatric bipolar can also be present in conjunction with Asperger's disorder. Typically, this is the case. It is unknown, however, if the pediatric bipolar disorder is a result of the Asperger's disorder, or if the same neurological issues that cause Asperger's disorder are related to the chemical imbalances in the brain thought to be the cause of pediatric bipolar disorder. Answers to these questions will likely come to light as research in neurological, technological and psychiatric areas continue to progress.

Medication treatments for pediatric bipolar and Asperger's disorders are quite similar. There are no medications for Asperger's disorder; however, medications exist to treat the symptoms of Asperger's disorder. Since the symptoms of Asperger's disorder, such as depression, obsessive compulsive disorder, and anxiety, are the same symptoms often experienced with pediatric bipolar disorder, the medications used in both instances are the same.

Counseling treatments are also commonly used for both pediatric bipolar and Asperger's disorders, used in conjunction with medication or alone. Most Asperger's patients do not need medication. Counseling is required, however, to help the patient cope with their disability. Counseling treatments for pediatric bipolar disorder are considered necessary, with or without medication. These treatments can help the patient learn to recognize and correct irrational emotions or behavior.

If you notice your child exhibiting any of the behaviors mentioned in this article, you should contact your pediatrician, doctor, therapist, or other health care professional to obtain a proper diagnosis and start a viable treatment plan. Undiagnosed or untreated pediatric bipolar or Asperger's disorder can lead to

Bipolar Disorder Treatment

Bipolar disorder treatment is not new. Men of medicine were treating for it before they even knew what it was. Yet every year new medications and methodologies are added to the bipolar disorder treatment.

Although first recognized in the second century A.D., bipolar disorder has struggled as a diagnosis to become accepted. Bipolar disorder treatment up to and through the 1960's, if any, was usually comprised of either locking the patient away or leaving him or her to fend for him or herself.

In the 1970's manic-depression, as it was then called, began to become seen as an accepted diagnosis and therefore, bipolar disorder treatment began in earnest. At that time, laws were enacted and standards set to help those who sought bipolar disorder treatment.

In bipolar disorder treatment, the first thought may be the use of medications. They are, actually, a powerful tool in the management of the disorder. One only needs look at the vast array of medications that is available to see that medication has been extensively used in bipolar disorder treatment.

Lithium carbonate was the first major breakthrough in the medications for bipolar disorder treatment. It belongs to a class of medications called "mood stabilizers". These medications help to prevent or ease manic episodes. They also help to ward off the extremes of depression, such as suicide.

Bipolar disorder treatment may also include the use of other mood stabilizers that were originally used as anticonvulsants. These have been shown to have a great effect on mood. Some of these, such as valproic acid and carbamazepine, are tried and true. Lamotrigine, gabapentin, and topiramate have also been used for this purpose but not conclusively proven effective.

Caution must be taken in the use of antidepressant therapy as a part of bipolar disorder treatment. Mood stabilizers are usually tried first, because antidepressants can trigger manic episodes or rapid-cycling. If an antidepressant must be used, there are certain ones which are less likely to cause these problems. One of these is bupropion.

The treatment of psychotic symptoms has evolved quickly in modern times. At first, there were powerful anti-psychotics. The first of these were said to put the mind in a "mental strait-jacket". They virtually stopped all thought. They also had an intense side effect known as tardive dyskinesia. This causes permanent neurological damages. Researchers then were trying to find alternatives that would cause less, or even no, damage in bipolar disorder treatment.

Other anti-psychotics were tried, and found to have fewer neurological effects. The newest of these medications are actually relatively safe when used as prescribed. They are also very helpful in bipolar disorder treatment both in psychotic episodes and even in simple mania. Some of the newer ones are risperidone and olanzapine.

Talk therapy is also used in bipolar disorder treatment. It can be useful to help a person to recognize and deal with symptoms of the disorder. Cognitive behavioral therapy can help a person to identify destructive patterns of thinking and behavior, and help him or her to act in ways that will have a positive influence on his or her disease process.

Other types of talk therapy are used in bipolar disorder treatment to help a person to deal with the devastating consequences of the illness and to explore the history of that person's disease. Talk therapy has been used successfully in bipolar disorder treatment.

All of these components constitute a lifelong process. Medication and talk therapy can contribute to effective bipolar disorder treatment today. No one knows what science will bring to bipolar disorder treatment in the future.

Other Treatments for Bipolar Disorder

Bipolar disorder, or manic depression, is a mental illness which causes mood swings and mood cycling. Mood cycling refers to the transition between mania and depression. Mania, or manic episodes, typically consist of feelings of elation and invincibility, and cause disorientation, lack of sleep, and obsessive behaviors. Depression typically consists of feelings of overwhelming sadness and low self-worth.

There are many treatments available for bipolar disorder, ranging from medications to therapy. There are too many medications to be discussed here in depth. There are also many forms therapy can take, and techniques that can be learned to assist the patient in gaining some control over their bipolar disorder.

Typically, bipolar disorder is treated with more than one medication. This is due to the dual nature of bipolar disorder. Most patients need at least two medications: one to control depression and one to control mania. The combination of these two types of medication works to obtain balance in moods and stop mood cycling. Often, a third medication, called a mood stabilizer, is also prescribed. The most common mood stabilizer is Topomax.

Popular medications for treatment of mania in bipolar patients include lithium, valproate (Depakote), carbamazepine (Tegretol), olanzapine (Zyprexa), and ziprasidone (Geodon). Lithium has long been considered the miracle drug of bipolar disorder. It is a sodium based medication that helps to balance the chemical imbalance in the brain that causes manic episodes in bipolar patients.

Valproate, or Depakote, was originally developed as a seizure medication. However, its effects on bipolar patients who have rapid cycling bipolar (moods that cycle every few hours or days rather than weeks or months), it has been quite effective. Carbamazepine, or Tegretol, is another anti-seizure medication. While it appears to have similar effects on bipolar disorder as Depakote, it has not yet been approved by the Food and Drug Administration for use as a bipolar disorder treatment.

Olanzapine, or Zyprexa, and Ziprasidone, or Geodon, are both anti-psychotic drugs, and are particularly effective for treatment of bipolar disorder in which mania becomes so severe that psychotic symptoms are present.

Medications for treatment of depression are called anti-depressants. Common anti-depressants include citalopram (Celexa), escitalopram (Lexapro), fluoxetine (Prozac), paroxetine (Paxil), and sertraline (Zoloft). All of these medications have been proven to be successful treatments for depression, although Celexa and Prozac are the most commonly prescribed.

Typically, treatment of bipolar disorder includes a combination of medications and therapy, or counseling. However, in some cases, medication may not be necessary for milder cases of bipolar disorder. In other cases, medication may not be desired by the patient, and the patient may wish to seek out other alternatives to medication for treatment of their bipolar disorder.

For these patients, Cognitive Behavioral Therapy (CBT) can be quite effective. CBT is a method of bipolar disorder treatment that involves teaching the patient techniques to recognize triggers and symptoms of their mood cycling, and use that information and recognition to prevent the triggers from occurring, or the mood cycling from being quite as severe. Most of these techniques require the patient to develop cognitive thinking skills as well as critical thinking and problem solving capabilities. If the bipolar disorder is severe to the point that the patient is unable to engage in these thinking abilities and skills, CBT may not be a viable form of treatment in and of itself.

Overall, there are many treatments available for bipolar disorder. There are many options for the patient that can be discussed with the patient's doctors. If a patient is not satisfied with the form their treatment is taking, they should discuss it with their doctor, and not be afraid to change doctors in order to change treatment methods. All in all, effective and successful treatment of bipolar disorder rests in the hands of the patient.

Childhood Treatment Options

Bipolar disorder, or manic depression, has in past years only been found in adults, while children with similar symptoms have been mistakenly diagnosed as have attention deficit disorder (ADD), or attention deficit hyperactivity disorder (ADHD). However, in recent years, psychiatrists and pediatricians have found that bipolar disorder definitely rears its ugly head in childhood as often as it does in adolescent or adult years.

Diagnosis of bipolar in childhood increases the chances for bipolar patients to have successful treatment and ordinary, uninhibited lives as adults. However, treatment options of bipolar in childhood is a controversial subject. Many doctors wish to medicate first, and regulate with therapy in addition to medications. However, many parents and some psychologists disagree with these methods.

Overall, many parents discover that once their child has been put on bipolar medications, the child seems to lose some of their personality traits that endear them to the parents. Children, and adults, who have been overly medicated or medicated when not absolutely necessary lose a sense of who they are. Some medications can make children overly despondent, seeming "out of it" or "spacey." This causes concern for parents and doctors, and raises the question of whether or not the child is really better off on medication.

Play therapy can be quite effective in helping children with bipolar disorder live more successful childhoods. This play therapy typically involves placing children in various hypothetical situations in which they must work out a logical and emotionally healthy solution. While play therapy is very successful in some children, it is not enough for others. In certain childhood cases of bipolar disorder, the mood swings and symptoms are so severe that the child is not able to control their actions or emotional reactions to stimuli and situations.

Cognitive behavioral therapy is a fairly new method of therapy for bipolar patients in which the patient learns to recognize symptoms of their illness, triggers for mood swings and inappropriate behavior, and alternatives to inappropriate behavior. Cognitive behavioral therapy also allows the patient to discover what he or she can do to avoid manic or depressive episodes, and how to manage the episodes more effectively. In adults, this treatment option is very viable, and works well both in conjunction with and without medication treatment.

However, cognitive behavioral therapy requires a level of problem solving and critical thinking that is not often present in childhood. For this reason, it is not commonly used in children with bipolar disorder under a certain age or maturity level. Some believe that the techniques learned through cognitive behavioral therapy could be equally viable in treating childhood bipolar disorder if the exercises and learning could be geared toward children. This, however, could prove difficult.

In the end, treatment options must be discussed with pediatricians, psychiatrists, psychologists, parents, and teachers. Everyone involved in childhood must be involved in the treatment process in order for it to be successful. If a parent or teacher has concerns about the effects of childhood treatment for bipolar disorder in their child or student, those concerns should be expressed immediately so that changes in treatment can be made. Additionally, parents should not be afraid to change doctors if they feel their child is not benefiting from treatment or medication.

Latest Medications for Bipolar Affective Disorder

Bipolar affective disorder, also known as manic depression disorder, is a mental illness that causes the patient to experience mood swings or mood cycling, involving depressive episodes, mania episodes, and/or mixed episodes. There are many treatment options for bipolar affective disorder. The most successful treatments are a combination of medications and counseling or therapy.

Within the last five years there have been several substantial breakthroughs in research toward finding the true biological cause of bipolar affective disorder. This research has led to the development of several new bipolar affective disorder medications. A few of the more popular latest medications for bipolar affective disorder are described below.

Abilify, or Aripiprazole, is an atypical anti-psychotic. It was approved for treatment of manic and mixed bipolar disorder episodes in 2004, and further approved as a maintenance medication for bipolar disorder in 2005. While most anti-psychotic medications work by shutting down dopamine receptors in the brain, Abilify works by making the dopamine receptors behave more normally. This stabilization makes this latest medication the ideal treatment for bipolar affective disorder.

Celexa is an antidepressant that has been around for several years. However, it has been used with increasingly more frequency in the last few years for the treatment of bipolar affective disorder. This is due to the fact that Celexa has proven to be more selective than other anti-depressants. This essentially means that with Celexa, fewer bipolar patients need a mood stabilizer to prevent the antidepressant from sending them zooming into a manic episode. It has been extremely successful as a maintenance medication for bipolar affective disorder.

Geodon is an anti-psychotic that works as a mood stabilizer in bipolar affective disorder patients. The most exciting thing about this latest mood stabilizer medication is that it is not associated with weight gain. It works in much the same way as Zyprexa, which has been proven to be a very successful medication for the treatment of bipolar affective disorder. However, unlike Zyprexa, side effects are fewer, milder, and do not include weight gain!

Wellbutrin, also sold as Zyban, was originally developed as a medication to help people stop smoking, in which it has been quite successful. In recent years, however, it has been discovered, quite by accident, that it is even more successful as an antidepressant when used as a medication for bipolar affective disorder. Chemically, it is unrelated to any other antidepressant, and it is unknown why it works so well with bipolar patients. One advantage to Wellbutrin is that it is a weight stable medication, meaning that patients will typically not see weight gain or weight loss.

As technology and research progresses, more effective medications for bipolar affective disorder are bound to be developed. Successful treatment of bipolar affective disorder is the goal of many researchers, psychologists, and psychiatrists. Discuss treatment options with your doctor often, and keep track of the latest developments in medications for bipolar affective disorder, so that you can appreciate the benefits of successful treatment for your bipolar affective disorder.

CBT as Treatment for Bipolar Disorder

Bipolar disorder, known by many as manic depression, is a mental illness caused by a combination of factors, including neurological, biological, emotional, and environmental factors. It is most commonly described as mood cycling or mood swings, in which the patient cycles through moods of depression, mania, and normal behavior.

There are many treatment options for bipolar disorder. The most common treatment for bipolar disorder includes a combination of medication and therapy. However, some patients are not candidates for medication treatment. Patients that have a history of drug abuse, for instance, should in most cases not be placed on medication for bipolar disorder, as the risk for abuse is too great. Additionally, patients may not have a case of bipolar disorder severe enough to warrant medication. Other patients may choose to avoid the route of medication until it becomes absolutely necessary.

In response to these special cases in which medication treatment is not a viable option for bipolar disorder, that Cognitive Behavioral Therapy, or CBT, was developed. CBT is a type of therapy that assists patients in recognizing triggers and causes for their manic and depressive states. The patient can then learn techniques to avoid these triggers, and cope with symptoms during episodes. Seventy percent of bipolar disorder type one patients that undergo CBT experience one or fewer episodes within four years of starting the CBT treatment.

There are two main goals that are met by using CBT as treatment for bipolar disorder. The first goal is to recognize manic episodes before they become uncontrollable, and consciously change how they react to the episode. The second goal is to learn techniques, reactions, thoughts, and behaviors that can help to offset depression. These goals are realized through various techniques and activities prescribed by the therapist. With CBT, the treatment of bipolar disorder rests with the patient, who is given homework in the form of exercises and reading, which helps them to understand their condition and learn methods to cope with it.

The first step to successful treatment of bipolar disorder through CBT is to develop a treatment contract with the patient. This is a treatment plan that the patient agrees to follow, and also involves the patient's promise to complete all homework assignments and take any prescribed medication as directed. Because the success of CBT depends largely on the patient's responsibility and desire to cope with bipolar disorder, this is an important first step to successful treatment.

The second step to successful treatment of bipolar disorder through CBT is to monitor and grade moods. This is done with various worksheets that the therapist gives the patient. The patient may record their mood for the day, how many hours they have slept, their level of anxiety, and their level of irritability. Those with type two bipolar disorder may need to record their mood two or more times per day, as their moods cycle more often.

Understanding the pattern to mood cycling can help the patient then undergo the next step to CBT treatment for bipolar disorder. This step of CBT for treatment of bipolar disorder requires the patient to do homework in the form of worksheets and reading that will help the patient to understand how their thoughts effect their emotions. By understanding these things, the patient will be able to then practice altering their thoughts in a rational way to make emotions more rational as well, decreasing the number and severity of depressive and manic episodes.

The next step to CBT treatment for bipolar disorder is to learn how to recognize triggers. Triggers are the thoughts, emotions, situations, times of year, events, or environments that set off a depressive or manic episode. By learning how to understand and recognize their triggers, the patient can then learn to avoid the triggers entirely, thereby decreasing the number and severity of depressive and manic episodes.

Overall, CBT is a viable and quite successful treatment for bipolar disorder, and can be a healthy alternative to medication in some cases. If you feel you may be a candidate for CBT, you should contact your doctor or therapist to discuss this and other bipolar disorder treatment options.

Made in the USA
Lexington, KY
06 November 2012